Blood Pressure

A Naturopathic Approach

Jane Semple, MA, ND

WOODLAND PUBLISHING

For permissions, ordering information, or bulk quantity discounts, contact: Woodland Publishing, 448 East 800 North, Orem, Utah 84097

Visit our Web site: www.woodlandpublishing.com
Toll-free number: (800) 777-2665

The information in this book is for educational purposes only and is not recommended as a means of diagnosing or treating an illness. All matters concerning physical and mental health should be supervised by a health practitioner knowledgeable in treating that particular condition. Neither the publisher nor the author directly or indirectly dispenses medical advice, nor do they prescribe any remedies or assume any responsibility for those who choose to treat themselves.

Cataloging-in-Publication data is available from the Library of Congress.

ISBN 978-1-58054-107-7

Printed in the United States of America

Contents

According to the USDA, the annual economic impact of cardio-vascular disease in the United States exceeds $80 billion. Conventional medicine has a tendency to isolate single disease characteristics like blood pressure or cholesterol, and look to drugs for treatment. There is rarely a single factor responsible for elevated blood pressure (hypertension) or low blood pressure (hypotension).

Multiple body systems work hand-in-hand to regulate blood pressure. How fast the heart beats, the force of contraction, and the flexibility of the arteries has a great deal to do with blood pressure. However, blood pressure control does not end within the circulatory system.

Many natural-health practitioners consider the digestive system to be the master system, as digestion and assimilation is where health begins. Food allergies and caffeine are known to increase heart rate. What we eat and drink affects blood pressure, as will be discussed throughout this book.

The nephron is the work center of the kidneys. Filtration occurs as fluid similar to blood plasma is pushed through the nephron where it sorts through, deciding what to keep, like amino acids and glucose (sugar), and what to release with the urine, like toxic byproducts of metabolism and excess minerals. If blood pressure is low, nephron pressure will be low and will not allow sufficient filtration. The nephron will signal the release of renin to increase blood pressure so that the kidneys can function properly.

Several glands play a part in blood pressure regulation. The pituitary gland regulates blood pressure through release of vasopressin, an antidiuretic hormone. The adrenal gland, which sits atop the kidney, targets the kidney to balance sodium, potassium and water. The thyroid gland assists in regulation of the rate and force of contraction of the heart.

Most people with blood pressure problems are concerned their blood pressure is too high, which will be the main focus of this book. However, those suffering from low blood pressure, hypotension, may also find the answer here.

How High Is "High"?

According to the *Current Medical Diagnosis and Treatment* (CMDT), the physician's bible, the following are recommendations for systolic and diastolic blood pressure. For simplicity, 120 mm Hg will simply be referred to as 120.

- Below 120/80 is optimal
- Below 130/85 is normal
- Between 130/85 and 139/90 is high normal
- Between 140/90 and 159/99 is stage 1 (mild)
- Between 160/100 and 179/109 is stage 2 (moderate)
- Higher than 180/110 is stage 3 (severe)

Blood pressure should be taken in a seated position, back supported, resting comfortably for a minimum of five minutes, and 30 minutes after smoking or drinking a caffeinated beverage.

Hypertension is diagnosed based upon elevation of either systolic or diastolic blood pressure. A diagnosis of hypertension should be made based on multiple readings taken over several days.

We do blood pressure readings in my office. When I get a reading that is slightly high, I say, "that's pretty good, let's do one more." The second reading is usually lower. I used to say, "that's a little high, let's do one more," and the second reading was nearly always higher. I suggest that my clients who have been diagnosed based on physician office readings to purchase a good blood pressure machine and track their own pressure. If your physician insists that the reading in their office is the only one that counts, then get a new physician, as this is more related to ego than concern for your well-being.

People with daytime average pressure of less than 135/85 have a low rate of cardiovascular complications and a low prevalence of left ventricular hypertrophy (discussed later). Fifty million Americans have blood pressure above 140/90, but only 50 percent take prescription medication. Hypertension increases with age and is more prevalent in blacks than whites. In people over the age of 50, systolic pressure is a better predictor of complications than diastolic pressure. (CMDT)

According to the CMDT, continued hypertension does not necessarily indicate the need for drug treatment. Assessment of the risk/benefit ratio of drug therapy should be done for patients with stage 1 hypertension (159/99). Physicians are highly variable on their opinions regarding blood pressure. I have clients with moderate hypertension where their physician gives them the option of whether or not to take a drug. Other physicians are quick to write a prescription for mild elevations.

I had a client with a history of blood pressure readings below 120/80. She had a single reading in her physician's office of 135/85, so he immediately put her on a prescription drug. She came to me with dizzy spells and extreme fatigue. I did two blood pressure readings during her afternoon consultation, one was 90/60, the second was 87/59. Her dizziness and fatigue were likely due to her blood pressure being too low. She had reported her symptoms and low blood pressure to her physician, but he "would not let her go off the medication." Just because a drug is prescribed, does not mean you have to take it. *There really is no law!* Too much of my time is taken up explaining that physicians are not even following their own guidelines!

Systolic and diastolic blood pressure tend to go together; for example, 100/70, 120/80 or 140/90. When this is true, a diagnosis of hypertension is easy. However, as people age, systolic pressure often rises out of proportion to diastolic; for example, 120/60, 140/65 or 180/80.

Many years ago, conventional wisdom was that systolic blood pressure should be not more than "100 plus your age." Thus a 60-year-old should have systolic pressure of no higher than 160; an 80-year-old should have systolic pressure of no higher than 180.

One 85-year-old client came in with blood pressure of 170/73. Her physician prescribed hydrochlorothiazide (a diuretic), atenolol (a beta-blocker) and verapamil (a calcium channel blocker). These three drugs together brought her blood pressure down to 154/67, leaving her barely able to breathe or walk. Within two weeks of starting the drugs, she stopped all of them. I suggested walking, elimination of a few trigger foods based on her blood type, and adding magnesium and hawthorn berries. It has been three years (yes, she is 88), and her last three drug-free blood pressure readings were 154/68, 157/56 and 148/61—excellent for her age.

A 62-year-old woman had moderately high pressure of 160/90, for which her physician prescribed a calcium channel blocker. She was upset because one of the side effects of calcium channel blockers is heart failure. This woman has a family history of females living well into their 90s. A calcium channel blocker would likely put someone into heart failure long before thirty years. When she exercised, her pressure would drop to 140/85 for 24 to 48 hours; a very reasonable pressure. However, she could not seem to find the time to exercise more than two days a week. I suggested three days of exercise per week or drugs—her choice.

I never suggest that someone should ignore truly high blood pressure. Many people schedule a consultation with me because they think I have a magic pill to replace their drugs. Some are not too happy to find out that I recommend exercise, diet, moderate weight loss and supplements. When people come back week after week with no change in pressure, I ask, are you exercising? No. Are you following the diet? No. Have you lost any weight? No. Then get back on your drugs because I cannot help you.

Why Be Concerned When Your Blood Pressure Is Too High?

High blood pressure strains the heart. Left ventricular hypertrophy is found in up to 15 percent of people with longstanding hypertension. Hypertrophy is where an organ, or in this case the left side of the heart, enlarges to compensate for increased demand or valve disorder. Enlargement may lead to heart failure or sudden death.

High blood pressure increases the risk of stroke, especially intracerebral hemorrhage (bleeding in the brain). Stroke complications are associated with severely elevated systolic pressure.

High blood pressure increases nephron pressure in the kidneys. The kidneys can safely excrete amino acids, but proteins (strings of amino acids) are too large. When pressure is too high, proteins are pushed through, damaging the nephron and thus the kidneys. When sufficient nephrons have sustained damage, a person is considered to be in kidney failure.

What Conventional Medicine Has to Offer

Conventional physicians have an array of pharmaceutical drugs they can prescribe for hypertension. It is interesting that the possible side effects of these drugs are similar to the damage expected from long-term blood pressure elevation.

Diuretics

Diuretics are divided into three groups:

1. Loop diuretics include bumetanide/Bumex, ethacrynate/ethacrynic/Edecrin, furosemide/Lasix/Novosemide/Uritol, and torsemide/Demadex.

2. Potassium-sparing diuretics include amiloride/Midamor, spironolactone/Aldactone, and triamterene/Dyrenium.

3. Hydrochlorothiazide is a thiazide diuretic. Brand names include Apo-Hydro, Diuchlor H, Esidrix, Hydro-chlor, Hydro-D, HydroDiuril, Neo-Codema, Novo-Hydrazide, Oretic and Urozide.

Diuretics act on the kidneys to eliminate sodium and water, thus reducing blood volume. This class of drugs may cause an imbalance in important electrolytes, including sodium, potassium or magnesium, leading to irregular heart rhythms. Other adverse reactions include elevated blood glucose levels, nausea, vomiting, headache, weakness, fatigue, constipation, cough and breathing difficulties. Diuretics should be used cautiously, if at all, by people with kidney or liver dysfunction.

Angiotensin-converting Enzyme (ACE) Inhibitors

Angiotensin-converting enzyme (ACE) inhibitors include benazepril/Lotensin, captopril/Capoten, enalapril/Vasotec, fosinopril/Monopril, lisinopril/Prinivil/Zestril, moexipril/Univasc, perindopril/Aceon, quinapril/Accupril, ramipril/Altace and trandolapril/Mavik.

ACE inhibitors reduce the release of angiotensin. You may recall that when nephron pressure in the kidneys is low, the kidney releases renin. Renin acts on angiotensin to raise nephron pressure and blood pressure. Angiotensin constricts blood vessels, so inhibiting its release would relax blood vessels.

Common adverse effects of ACE inhibitors are headache, fatigue, tachycardia (fast heartbeat), taste perversion, protein in the urine, high potassium, rash, cough, as well as swelling of face and limbs. Protein in the urine is an indication of kidney damage, which may lead to kidney failure. Potassium is needed for the electrical conduction of heart and nerve impulses. ACE inhibitors may reduce the number of white blood cells, impairing immune function.

ACE inhibitors have long been cautioned in the last two trimesters of pregnancy due to possible kidney damage or malformation of the fetus. However, newer research reports this class of drugs is also dangerous during the first trimester, causing fetal defects of the heart, limbs, brain and spinal cord. ACE inhibitors can cause permanent disability and retardation. (Cooper, 2006) I recommend that every woman who is pregnant or planning to become pregnant work with a qualified alternative health practitioner to minimize the use of prescription drug through diet and lifestyle. If you must take prescription drugs during pregnancy, dosage should be at the absolute minimum.

Beta Blockers

Beta blockers used to treat hypertension include acebutolol/Sectral, atenolol/Tenormin, betaxolol/Betoptic/Kerlone, bisoprolol/ Zebeta, esmolol/Brevibloc, and metoprolol/Toprol/Lopressor.

Although the exact mechanism of action is unknown, this pharmaceutical class decreases cardiac output, slows the heart, and suppresses renin release. I can usually tell when a client is on a beta-blocker, as their heart rate is unusually low.

Side effects include bradycardia (slow heartbeat), fatigue, dizziness, nightmares, depression, memory loss, hallucinations, cold limbs, elevated cholesterol levels, heart failure and impotence.

Calcium Channel Blockers

Calcium channel blockers include amlodipine/Norvasc, diltiazem/ Cardizem/Dilacor/Tiazac, felodipine/Plendil, isradipine/DynaCirc, nicardipine/Cardene, nifedipine/Adalat/Procardia, nimodipine/ Nimotop, nisoldipine/Sular, and verapamil/Calan/Isoptin/Verelan.

Calcium channel blockers inhibit the influx of calcium, relaxing the muscles and dilating blood vessels. Side effects include bradycardia, heart attack, heart block, worsening heart failure, irregular heartbeat, shortness of breath, swelling of hands and feet, pronounced dizziness, constipation, nausea and liver damage.

When I was taking a conventional medical pharmacology class, we were cautioned to reserve calcium channel blockers for elderly patients. This was due to the high rate of heart failure caused by this class of drugs. What constitutes an elderly patient? Some young physicians consider anyone over 65 to have one foot in the grave. I look at the longest-lived relatives, especially on the mother's side and subtract ten years.

What Nature Has to Offer

I insist on doing a full workup with regular follow-up for anyone with moderate to severe hypertension (above 160/100). If you are in this group, you may be able to reduce your medication by following several of my suggestions. Do not reduce your medication dosage until natural measures are working.

If your blood pressure is high normal or moderately high, then diet, lifestyle and supplements may keep it within normal range, without the need for drug therapy. Since there is no single cause of elevated blood pressure, there is no single magic bullet. Please monitor your blood pressure regularly.

Keep in mind, our blood pressure tends to increase as we age. Do not be overly concerned with a slight elevation if you are over 70, unless you have been diagnosed with cardiovascular disease or have an underlying illness like uncontrolled diabetes.

Elevated blood pressure indicates something is wrong. Drugs do not deal with the cause. It is not lowering blood pressure, but *how* you lower blood pressure that will both add years to your life and life to your years.

Exercise

Even modest increases in exercise can reduce blood pressure. Walk, join a spa or a gym, whatever your preference. Increase your general activity level. When watching television, walk up and down the stairs during commercials. If your house is full of clutter, put a few things away during commercials. You are not missing anything except a bunch of commercials for drugs you do not need.

Some clients claim they can't exercise because their knees hurt or some other excuse. If a person in a wheelchair can exercise, then someone with a bad knee can exercise. Do chair exercises if you need to. See an exercise physiologist who can set up a program for you.

Diet

Eat seven servings of vegetables and fruit per day at the very minimum. One-half cup of vegetables is a serving. A small apple is a serving, while most apples today are two servings. Corn and white pota-toes (regardless of skin color) are not vegetables for our purposes.

Water retention has been related to binge eating of carbohydrates and sodium after a period of near fasting. (MacGregor, 1979) I find a diet high in vegetables with some fruit and lean meat and limited carbohydrates reduces water retention, which in turn reduces blood pressure.

I have had a great deal of success with the book *Eat Right for Your Type* by Dr. Peter D'Adamo. D'Adamo's work is based on decades of research into the way various foods react with blood antigens. A client purchases his or her blood type booklet on their first visit.

In general, A's do best with lots of vegetables and fruit along with turkey, chicken and some fish. Blood type A's will have problems when they eat too many animal products, especially pork, beef and cheese.

One client went on the Atkins diet. She lost weight, but her cho-lesterol and blood pressure rose significantly. Atkins is too high in animal products for blood type A's.

I was counseling a young man with blood type A. As I was explain-ing what he should and should not eat, he said that is exactly how he ate before he was married, and his blood pressure was fine.

Blood type B's do best with lots of vegetables along with lamb and game meat like rabbit and venison. B's can also eat beef, turkey, some fish and some dairy products, avoiding pork, chicken and corn.

One type-B client could not control his blood pressure. He came to me when his physician prescribed drugs, which he refused to take. This client was overweight, did not exercise, was eating excessive chicken (an avoid), and his favorite meal was lobster (an avoid) cooked in a broth of corn (an avoid). I counseled him on portion control and exercise, as he was already taking a significant number of supplements, though not specifically related to blood pressure. The following year, his blood pressure was higher. He had gained weight, was not exercising, and not following the blood type diet. I advised him to do drugs!

Type O's do best with vegetables along with meat, with the excep-tion of pork. In addition to avoiding pork, blood type O's should avoid kidney and navy beans, diary products, corn and wheat.

I consulted with a fifteen-year-old client with a blood pressure of 140/90. Her physician wanted to put her on an ACE inhibitor. Her father, in his 40s, had been on blood pressure drugs since his late teens and was now nearing kidney failure. The physician assumed the girl "inherited" high blood pressure. I said she inherited her father's blood type and eating habits. When discussing what D'Adamo called "avoid foods," I hit a nerve when I mentioned corn. When this girl stopped eating corn, her blood pressure fell to 90/60 within a week! That was several years ago, and her blood pressure continues to be normal as long as she follows her blood type diet.

If your blood pressure is high and you do not find something you are eating excessively in this list, please get a copy of *Eat Right for Your Type* and search the food lists. I find that the younger the client, the quicker their blood pressure normalizes. In clients over age 70, the damage is likely done, though the blood type diet can still offer a moderate reduction.

Water

Insufficient water leading to dehydration is a major factor in blood pressure control, contributing to both hypertension and hypotension. Dehydration is also a major factor in stroke and atrial fibrillation.

Several years ago, I was teaching a class when I stated that dehydration could cause atrial fibrillation. A man in the class had gone to the ER several months before with atrial fib, which converted to normal sinus rhythm once he was put on IV fluids while waiting for a physician.

In a more recent class, I was relaying this story. A registered nurse in the class often worked in a cardiac unit. The following week, she converted five out of seven patients from atrial fib to normal sinus rhythm simply by turning up the IV drip, which rehydrated the patient more quickly.

Things you can do in addition to exercise, diet and ensuring adequate water intake:

- Keep weight within normal range. Obesity is associated with hypertension.
- If you smoke, stop. Cigarette smoking raises blood pressure by increasing levels of norepinephrine.
- Keep alcohol consumption below two drinks daily for men and one drink for women. Avoid binge drinking.
- Reduce sodium intake and increase potassium intake. The sodium/potassium ratio is particularly important. Herbs and vegetables tend to be especially high in potassium.
- Estrogen usually results in a small increase in blood pressure. However, in some women, birth control pills or hormone replacement used in menopause cause a considerable rise. Be aware of this possibility and monitor blood pressure regularly.
- NSAIDs like Advil, Aleve, Motrin, Celebrex and others increase blood pressure. If you take NSAIDs regularly for any condition, please see a naturopath or herbalist for recommendations to treat the underlying cause.

Herbs and Supplements for Blood Pressure Regulation

Chelating Agents

Oral chelation supplements are specially formulated to provide high-dose nutrients to clear arteries. I find oral chelation helpful for lowering blood pressure in addition to reducing cholesterol and inflammation. Naturopaths use oral chelation, rather than invasive intravenous chelation. IVs are expensive, and, in my opinion, rarely necessary.

Oral chelation starts with low-dose supplements, increasing over several weeks until the maximum dosage is attained. The rule of thumb is to stay at the higher dose one month for every ten years of life. Supplements are increased for one month, then tapered off for one month.

Thus, a 50-year-old person would be on a program for seven

months. One month of increasing dosage, five months at maximum dosage, then one month tapering off. A 70-year-old person would be on a program for a total of nine months. Keep in mind that maximum dosages are usually given for adult men. Dosages should be reduced for women based on height and build, not just total weight.

For a serious problem, I recommend the full program be repeated yearly. For a less serious problem, a three-month program repeated yearly may be sufficient.

Your naturopath or herbalist should be able to guide you through a chelation program. If you are on an excessive number of drugs or are diagnosed with serious heart disease, please work with a knowledgeable practitioner.

Cayenne

Cayenne (*Capsicum annuum*) is hot red pepper, which stimulates blood flow and strengthens the heartbeat. (Henry and Emery, 1986) Cayenne improves peripheral circulation, blood flow to the extremities. (Glatzel, 1967)

Cayenne regulates blood pressure up or down as necessary, and may prevent heart attack and stroke. An extract has been used sublingually (under the tongue) in mild to moderate heart attacks.

In a three-year study of 920 patients, the death rate among patients suffering mild heart attacks was one-third higher among those receiving aggressive treatment with invasive procedures including angiography, angioplasty and bypass surgery compared to those receiving only drugs and supportive therapy. (Bolen, 1997)

I have several die-hard herbal clients who consider hospitals to be death traps and have ridden out a series of mild heart attacks, much to their physician's dismay. I suggest a squirt of capsicum extract, under the tongue, repeated every few minutes until the sensation eases. Each person has reported back that it works. A few women use it regularly.

I suggest capsicum to my patients who have gone to the ER on one or two occasions and have been told it is simply indigestion. They do not want to spend hours at an ER, at great expense, for no purpose. The capsicum extract works for them as well.

Garlic

Garlic (*Allium sativum*): According to Mark Blumenthal of the American Botanical Council, by 1996 there were over 1,800 scientific studies showing garlic as beneficial to the cardiovascular system. Published studies include 96 on blood pressure, 69 on coagulation and flow and 82 on platelet aggregation.

An eight-week study reduced blood pressure in 47 people from an average of 171/102 to 155/91 (Auer, 1990). A four-year clinical trial of garlic found a 9–18 percent reduction in plaque, and a 7 percent lowering of blood pressure. The reduction of blood pressure was assumed to be due to an opening of calcium ion channels in the smooth muscle of blood vessels. Vascular diameter increased 4 percent. Reduction of stroke and infarction was greater than 50 percent. (Siegel, 1999)

Numerous studies have shown smaller, but consistent, positive effects of garlic on blood pressure. I do not recommend garlic as the sole treatment unless blood pressure is only slightly elevated. If blood pressure is low, garlic will not reduce it further. I like to use a combination of capsicum with garlic to regulate blood pressure. I recommend this combination to clients with slightly elevated blood pressure as well as those whose pressure tends to run a little low, especially in the afternoon.

Hawthorn Berry

Hawthorn berry (*Crataegus laevigata*) is approved by German Commission E for use in angina, arrhythmias and to improve cardiac muscle tone and circulation. Hawthorn has a long history of use for cardiovascular complaints, confirmed safety, and clinical evidence to support its benefits.

An ACE inhibitor is often the first drug of choice to lower blood pressure. Hawthorn inhibits angiotensin-converting enzymes, which is the mechanism of action of ACE inhibitors. (Uchida, 1987)

Heart failure is a problem in a small number of people with sustained elevated blood pressure. Studies with early stage congestive heart failure using dose ranges from 160 to 900 mg, showed impro-

ved heart function and exercise tolerance, and a lessening of shortness of breath and post-exercise fatigue. (Reuter, 1994; Zapfe, 1998)

Schultz cites 14 clinical studies published from 1981 to 1994 on
the therapeutic efficacy of hawthorn. Study participants included a
total of 808 patients with early congestive heart failure.

I recommend hawthorn or a combination of hawthorn with capsicum and garlic for clients with a personal or family history of cardiovascular disease. I take this combination myself because my
blood pressure runs a little low (100/70), but may drop to 90/60 or
below in the afternoon. I know it seems inconceivable that an herbal
combination can lower high blood pressure and raise low blood
pressure, but this combination does just that. Herbs tend to help the
body adapt by providing needed nutrients for self-regulation.

Calcium and Magnesium

Magnesium may reduce blood pressure by dilating the arteries. This
mineral prevents platelet aggregation and arrhythmias. Dr.
Zwilinger, a German physician, was the first to show the value of
magnesium in correcting arrhythmias in 1935. Several types of
blood medications, including diuretics and ACE inhibitors, may
deplete magnesium.

Calcium is the contractor, whereas magnesium is the relaxer. Calcium intake that is out of line with magnesium intake may cause
coronary heart disease. A U. S. study of 14,000 people followed for
seven years concluded that low magnesium levels contribute to the
origin of coronary atherosclerosis and acute heart attack. (Liao,
1998)

The Centers for Disease Control and Prevention in Atlanta followed 12,000 people for nineteen years. Researchers made a conser-
vative estimate that 11 percent of people dying of heart disease could
have been directly related to magnesium deficiency. (Ford, 1999)

Dr. James Pierce believes angina that occurs at rest is directly related to low magnesium levels, and estimates that up to 50 percent of
sudden heart attacks may be due to magnesium deficiency. He found
that magnesium worked better than nitroglycerine for his own

stress-induced chest pain. *Note: a capsule of magnesium may be opened and poured under the tongue, where many blood vessels are located. This gets the mineral into the circulatory system quickly.*

When a client schedules an appointment with me, my staff instructs the client to bring in any herbs, vitamins and minerals they are currently taking. Clients are instructed to bring the bottles, not a list. I am no longer surprised to find calcium with no magnesium to balance it. This is especially true for menopausal women, where their physician has recommended high doses of calcium to ward off osteoporosis.

Calcium is the contractor, allowing your heart to have a good, strong beat. Calcium contracts the blood vessels so the blood can be pushed through. Magnesium is the relaxer, allowing the heart muscle and arteries to relax between beats. I consider calcium alone to have a potential of raising blood pressure. I have seen blood pressure drop by 20 points when 500 to 1,000 mg of magnesium is added daily.

With magnesium, or any mineral, more is not always better. I had a client who was a little boy with a magnesium deficiency based on blood tests run by his physician. The physician recommended an excessive dose of magnesium powder, which caused extreme diarrhea, but did not raise his blood levels of this important mineral. I recommended his mother reduce the dosage. The diarrhea stopped and his blood magnesium levels rose to normal limits. When the digestive system is inundated with too much, even of a good thing, it will throw it off rather than assimilate it.

Potassium

Potassium is needed for electrical conduction of the heart. A potassium deficiency may exist despite normal blood potassium levels. Potassium deficiency is associated with heart arrhythmias as well as decreased tolerance to cardiac medications and EKG alterations. (Kafka, 1987; Nordrehaug, 1985) Potassium may be depleted by several blood pressure medications, especially thiazide diuretics and ACE inhibitors.

A study was conducted with 297 patients with congestive heart failure on diuretic therapy. Potassium losses caused low intracellular (within the cell) potassium. Magnesium loss led to further loss of intracellular potassium, as magnesium is necessary for proper functioning of the cell's calcium/potassium pump. Low potassium and magnesium caused elevated sodium in the heart muscle, while sodium levels in the blood were reduced. (Webster, 1980). Blood tests for minerals are not always an indicator of the actual mineral content of the heart or other tissue.

Since magnesium is necessary to get potassium into the cell, replacing potassium doesn't help patients who are also magnesium deficient, because the body is unable to deliver potassium into the cells. Magnesium and potassium are more effective when administered together due to the inability of the heart muscle to hold on to potassium in the absence of magnesium.

The potassium to sodium ratio may be more important than potassium alone. Most herbs and vegetables have good potassium to sodium ratios. Some herbs that are particularly high in potassium include kelp, dulse, alfalfa, horseradish and horsetail.

The amino acid 1-arginine is a precursor to nitric oxide, which supports normal blood pressure, heart function and male sexual function. Nitric oxide, formerly known as endothelium-derived relaxation factor, is a vasodilator, which means it relaxes or "opens" up the arteries. Arginine is found in meat, especially red meat, and chocolate.

I have found an occasional client who has responded quickly to 1-arginine supplementation. The client is likely a blood type O or blood type B who cut red meat out of their diet. If this amino acid does not reduce blood pressure within a few days, elevated blood pressure is not likely due to a shortage of 1-arginine. An ounce or two of dark chocolate daily is also a potential remedy.

Many people with high blood pressure have a personal or family history of cardiovascular disease. In addition to the major supplements covered, many supplements play a supporting role in cardiovascular disease, even though they may not have a drastic affect on blood pressure.

Dr. Peter Mitchell was awarded the Nobel Prize in Medicine in 1975 for his work on coenzyme Q10 (CoQ10, ubiquinone). An article reviewed 30 years of research on the use of CoQ10 in prevention and treatment of cardiovascular disease. This antioxidant has potential for use in prevention and treatment of high blood pressure, high cholesterol, coronary artery disease and heart failure. Cholesterol drugs, beta-blockers and some diabetic drugs reduce the level of CoQ10 in the body. The reviewer recommended CoQ10 supplementation as an adjunct to conventional treatment. (Sarter, 2002) When an important nutrient is so clearly depleted by a drug, the drug should be administered with extreme caution. If drug treatment is absolutely necessary, the nutrient should be replenished.

An Australian study followed 74 type 2 diabetics for 12 weeks. Patients were randomly assigned 200 mg of CoQ10 or fenobirate (fibric acid derivative used to reduce triglyceride levels). Both helped control blood glucose, but only CoQ10 additionally reduced blood pressure. CoQ10 reduced systolic pressure by an average of 6 points, and diastolic by an average of 3 points. (Hodgson, 2002)

Heart tissue levels of CoQ10 from 43 cardiomyopathy patients were biopsied. Deficiencies of this important coenzyme were directly related to severity of disease. The researchers concluded that CoQ10 is an effective treatment for cardiomyopathy. (Folkers, 1985)

CoQ10 (120 mg) was given to 73 patients with 71 in a control group. All patients had a recent myocardial infarction. In one year, the total number of cardiac events was 25 percent in the CoQ10 group, and 45 percent in the control group. Events included nonfatal infarction, 14 percent in CoQ10 group and 25 percent in the control group. Fatigue was reported by 7 percent of the CoQ10 group compared to 41 percent of the control group. (Singh, 2003)

Animal studies have shown CoQ10 to be safe, with no toxicity, even at extremely high doses. Use caution in withdrawing supplementation, as rebound may occur within a few weeks. Recommended dosages range between 30 mg and 300 mg daily.

Essential Fatty Acids

Essential fatty acids (EFAs) are healing fats. EFAs stimulate metabolism, increasing metabolic rate. EFAs are used as structural components of cell membranes and active body tissues (brain, nerve cells, retinas, adrenals, testes and ovaries). In addition, EFAs are used by enzymes and positively interact with proteins. (Erasmus)

Saturated fatty acids are solid at room temperature. They tend to stick together and cause cell membranes to become hard, choking off oxygen and reducing nutrient absorption by tissues.

The U. S. Department of Health and Human Services analyzed 123 studies that looked at omega-3's effect on risk factors and intermediate markers for cardiovascular disease. They found a small but significant reduction in both systolic and diastolic blood pressure. Three studies found that fish oil improved heart rate variability for patients with recent myocardial infarction. Fish oil has been found to increase exercise capability among patients with clogged arteries.

A reduction of blood pressure may be related to EFA's control of prostaglandins. "Bad" prostaglandins act as vasoconstrictors, narrowing blood vessels. EFAs then help the blood vessels to relax and expand.

Omega-3 fatty acids prevent further damage in men who have already had a heart attack, and may also prevent a first heart attack in both men and women. Fatty acids may stave off sudden cardiac death in people without signs of cardiovascular disease. (Hu, 2002)

A study reported in the *New England Journal of Medicine* followed healthy men for 17 years. The researchers found that omega-3s reduce risk of sudden death among men without evidence of prior cardiovascular disease. This is particularly important as more than 50 percent of all sudden deaths occur in people with no history of heart disease. (Albert, 2002)

The U. S. Department of Health and Human Services analyzed 39 omega-3 studies. Overall, the evidence shows that the consumption of omega-3 fatty acids (EPA, DHA), fish and fish oil reduce all-cause mortality and various cardiovascular disease outcomes such as heart attacks.

In a systematic review of evidence, the Agency for Healthcare Research and Quality (AHRQ) reported that fish oil reduced heart attacks and other problems related to heart and blood vessel disease. In addition, fish oil reduced the risk of reblockage after angioplasty.

According to Udo Erasmus in *Fats that Heal, Fats that Kill,* healing omega-3-containing foods (in order of best to good): flax oil, soybeans, fish, walnuts, seaweed, sunflower seeds, sesame seeds, almonds, borage oil, black currant oil and evening primrose oil. *Note: The last three oils are higher in gamma-linolenic omega-6 oil used by the adrenals and gonads.*

Oil-containing foods that can kill (from worst to bad): shortenings, margarine, frying oils, refined oils, pork, dairy products, roasted nuts and seeds.

Vitamin E

Vitamin E includes a group of related compounds including, d-alpha, -beta, -delta and gamma tocopherols and d-alpha, -beta, -delta and -gamma tocotrienols. The body does not recognize synthetic dl-alpha tocopherol.

Evan Shute, MD, a Canadian cardiologist was the first to document the cardiovascular benefits of vitamin E in the 1950s. He could not get published in the United States.

A study of U.S. nurses and doctors found a 30 to 40 percent reduction in the incidence of heart disease among those who had the highest level of vitamin E intake over an eight year period. The benefit was greatest in individuals taking more than 100 IU daily. (Diaz, 1997)

The U.S. Nurses' Health Study found a 34 percent reduction in cardiac mortality, and the U.S. Health Professional's Study found a 39 percent reduction in cardiac mortality in those who took daily vitamin E. The Iowa Women's Health Study and the Cambridge Heart Antioxidant Study found a 47 percent reduction in fatal and nonfatal heart attacks in patients with proven coronary disease taking 400 to 800 IU of vitamin E daily. Dr. David Emmert, who coauthored an article in the *Archives of Internal Medicine,* recommends 400 IU of vitamin E daily. (Emmert, 1999)

The National Cancer Institute, the American Heart Association and the United States Department of Agriculture endorse vitamin E supplementation.

A few recent studies suggest that supplemental vitamin E provides little benefit. Each negative study I have looked at used synthetic vitamin E (dl-tocopherol). I recommend 400 IU daily of a natural vitamin E (mixed tocopherols and tocotrienols) for those who choose to add this vitamin to their regimen.

Ginger

Ginger (*Zingiber officinale*) reduces platelet stickiness, which is one cause of stroke. The first time I donated platelets to the Red Cross, one of the technicians said my platelets were sticking, causing the machine to jam. She suggested the next time I donate I should take ginger the night before. I did and it worked!

If an herb used safely as a spice for thousands of years can do the job, and a blood bank technician is aware of its effects, why does a drug company see fit to develop an expensive drug, with a mountain of side effects, like clopidogrel/Plavix? Have ginger and Plavix gone toe to toe in a study? Of course not. Who would pay for it—the makers of Plavix? How about government-funded research—our hard-earned tax dollars that pay for a great deal of drug research.

A few years after I began to donate platelets, I decided if my platelets are sticky and ginger can keep them from sticking (one grandmother and one aunt died of stroke), then why not take ginger daily instead of just before a donation. I added one ginger capsule to my evening supplements.

How to Use this Book

If you have elevated blood pressure, please purchase a blood pressure machine and track your blood pressure several times per day. Your blood pressure is an average of several readings. Do not be concerned if one reading per day is high—just consider if a food allergy or stressful event may have caused it.

Do not reduce or stop prescription medications until diet and lifestyle changes along with supplements are working to reduce blood pressure. Supplements are more subtle than drugs in that they may take several days or weeks for you to notice a difference, so do not expect instant results.

I consider lifestyle changes and supplements to be a success if they allow you to reduce the number or dosage of drugs you are taking. Fewer drugs mean fewer side effects. Lower-dosage drugs mean reduced chance of side effects.

If you are concerned that you have to pay out of pocket for herbs, but your insurance pays for drugs, remember that we all pay for your drugs in higher insurance premiums. Diet and exercise that reduce blood pressure will improve health and lengthen life.

How to Locate a Practitioner

If your blood pressure is particularly high or if you have other factors that contribute to cardiovascular disease, look for a natural health-care practitioner near you. Check your local phone directory under Naturopaths, Herbs or Alternative Medicine. You may also contact the American Naturopathic Medical Association (ANMA), PO Box 96273, Las Vegas, NV 89193, www.anma.com. The ANMA is the oldest and largest naturopathic association, with approximately 4,000 members.

Bibliography

Agency for Healthcare Research and Quality. "Evidence reports confirm that fish oil helps fight heart disease." April 22, 2004.

Albert, C., H. Campos, M. Stampfer, et al. *New England Journal of Medicine*, vol. 346, April 11, 2002.

Alpert, Joseph, MD. *Cardiology for the Primary Care Physician.* St. Louis: Mosby, 1996.

Auer, W., et al. "Hypertension: garlic helps in mild cases." *British Journal Clinical Practice* 44 (supplement 69), 1990.

Barney, Paul, MD. *Doctor's Guide to Natural Medicine,* Orem, UT: Woodland Publishing, 1998.

Bland, Jeffrey, Ph.D. *Genetic Nutritioneering,* Los Angeles: Keats Publishing, 1999.

Blumenthal, Mark. *Clinical Guide to Herbs,* Austin: American Botanical Council, 2003.

Blumenthal, Mark, Alicia Goldberg and Josef Brickmann. *Herbal Medicine: Expanded Commission E Monographs.* Austin: American Botanical Council, 2000.

Bolen. American College of Cardiology, 1997.

Brown, D. *Herbal Prescriptions for Better Health.* Rocklin, CA: Prima Publishing, 1996.

Cooper, William, Sonia Hernandez-Diaz, et al. "Major congenital malformations after first-trimester exposure to ACE inhibitors." *New England Journal of Medicine,* vol. 354:2443–2451, June 8, 2006.

D'Adamo, Peter, ND. *Eat Right for Your Type.* New York: Putnam and Sons, 1996.

Dean, Carolyn, MD, ND. *Miracle of Magnesium,* Ballantine Books.

Diaz, M., B. Frei, et al. "Antioxidants and atherosclerotic heart disease." *New England Journal of Medicine,* No. 337, August 7, 1997.

Emmert, David, et al. "The role of vitamin E in the prevention of heart disease." *Archives of Family Medicine,* 8:537, December 3, 1999.

Erasmus, Udo. *Fats that Heal, Fats that Kill.* Burnaby, BC, Canada: Alive Books, 1993.

Folkers, Karl, et al. *Effective Therapy of Cardiomyopathy with Coenzyme Q10,* Procedures National Academy of Sciences, U.S.A., vol. 82:901, February 1, 1985.

Ford, Earl. "Serum magnesium and ischemic heart disease." *International Journal of Epidemiology,* vol. 28, 1999.

German Federal Institute for Drugs and Medical Devices Commission E, Blumenthal, et al. *Complete German Commission E Monographs,* Austin: American Botanical Council, 1998.

Glatzel, H. "Blood circulation effectiveness of natural products." *Medizinische Clinic,* (published in German), December 1967.

Goldberg, Burton. *Alternative Medicine Guide to Heart Disease, Stroke and High Blood Pressure,* Tiburon, CA: Future Medicine Publishing, 1998.

Henry, C. and B. Emery. "Effect of spiced food on metabolic rate." *Clinical Nutrition* 40:2, March 1986.

Herb Allure Resource Kit. Jamestown, NY: Herb Allure, 2004.

Hodgson, J., G. Watts, et al. "Coenzyme Q10 improves blood pressure: a controlled trial of subjects with type 2 diabetes." *European Journal of Clinical Nutrition,* 56(11):1137, November 2002.

Hu F., L. Bronner, et al. "Fish and Omega-3 fatty acid intake and risk of coronary heart disease in women," *JAMA,* 287:1815, April 10, 2002.

Koch, H. and L. Lawson. *Garlic: The Science and Therapeutic Application of Allium sativum.* Baltimore: Williams and Wilkins Publishing Co., 1996.

Langsjoen, P., S. Vadhanaviki, and K. Folkers. "Response of patients in class 3 and 4 of cardiomyopathy to therapy with Coenzyme Q10." *Proceedings of the National Academy of Sciences,* U.S.A. 82:4240, 1985.

Lawrence, Felicity. "Doctor's story exposes politics of research, profits," *Cleveland Plain Dealer,* May 29, 2000.

Liao, F., A. Folsom. "Is low magnesium concentration a risk factor for coronary heart disease?" *American Heart Journal,* vol. 136:3, 1998.

Lippicott, Williams and Wilkins. *Physician's Drug Handbook,* 11th Edition. Philadelphia, 2005.

Marchioli. "Dietary supplementation with n-3 fatty acids and vitamin E after myocardial infarction: results of GISSI-Prevention Trial." *Lancet,* 354:447, August 7, 1999.

Martini, Frederic. *Fundamentals of Anatomy and Physiology.* Upper Saddle River, NJ: Prentice Hall, 1995.

Morellia, Jim. "Is Vitamin E good for the heart?" WebMD Medical News Archive.

Muldoon, M., et al. University of Pittsburgh, *American Journal of Medicine,* May, 2000.

Nordrehaug. *Circulation* 71(4):645–49, 1985, 12.

Olszewski and McCully. *Coronary Artery Disease,* 1993.

Quillin, Patrick, Ph.D. *Beating Cancer with Nutrition.* Carlsbad, CA: Nutrition Times Press, 2001.

Reuter, H. *Hawthorn: A Botanical Cardiac Agent.* Z. Phytoher 15:73–81, 1994.

Sarter, B. "CoenzymeQ10 and cardiovascular disease: a review." *Journal of Cardiovascular Nursing,* 16(4):9–20, July 2002.

Singh, R., et al. "Effect of coenzyme Q10 on risk of atherosclerosis in patients with recent myocardial infarction." *Molecular and Cellular Biochemistry,* 246:75, April 2003.

Tierney, McPhee and Papadakis. *Current Medical Diagnosis and Treatment.* New York: McGraw Hill, Medical Publishing Division, 2004.

Twenty Essential Supplements for Super Health. Orem, UT: Woodland Publishing, 2005.

Uchida, S. *Japanese Journal of Pharmacology,* 43:242–5, 1987.

Verlangieri, A. Rutgers University, "The Riddle of Illness." Keats, 1984.

Webster, P. *Magnesium in Health and Disease.* Spectrum Publishing Company, 1980.

Werbach, Melvyn, MD. *Nutritional Influences on Illness.* Tarzana, CA: Third Line Press, 1996.

Zapfe, G., K. Assmus, H. Noh. "Placebo controlled multicenter study with hawthorn." Fifth Congress of Phytotherapy, Bonn, Germany, June 11, 1993.

Web Sites

American Botanical Council: www.herbalgram.org

U.S. Government Agency for Healthcare Research and Quality: www.ahrg.gov

Journal of the American Medical Association: www.jama.ama-assn.org

Medscape: www.medscape.com

New England Journal of Medicine: www.nejm.org

WebMD: www.webmd.com

About the Author

Dr. Jane Semple received her master's degree from Case Western Reserve, graduating first in her class in 1984. She completed a dual Doctorate in Naturopathy and Naturopathic Ministry from Trinity College of Natural Health. She has been an herbalist and naturopathic practitioner for twenty years.

Dr. Semple was a professor at Cuyahoga Community College for six years and Baldwin-Wallace College for three years. She developed an Anatomy and Physiology module for Trinity College of Natural Health.

She founded the Alternative Healing Institute to bring training for alternative therapies to individuals and medical professionals. She develops and teaches Continuing Education courses for those in the medical field.

Dr. Semple is an active member of the American Naturopathic Medical Association, the Association of Nutritional Consultants, American Botanical Council and Coalition for Natural Health. She is a Health Freedom advocate.

She has been listed in *Who's Who of American Women* since 1985, and *Who's Who in Medicine and Healthcare* since 2004. She was honored as a Woman of Achievement in Ohio in April 2005.

Other Books by the Author in the Woodland Health Series

Alzheimer Disease: A Naturopathic Approach

Cholesterol and Inflammation: A Naturopathic Approach

Fertility: A Naturopathic Approach

HPV and Cervical Dysplasia: A Naturopathic Approach

Influenza: Epidemics, Pandemics and the Bird Flu

Parkinson Disease: A Naturopathic Approach